Management of Peripheral Nerve Injuries and Role of Tendon Transfer

Management of Peripheral Nerve Injuries and Role of Tendon Transfer

Vishwa Prakash MS, MCh
Chief of third unit of Plastic Surgery
Safdarjung hospital and
VM Medical College
New Delhi

PEEPEE
PUBLISHERS & DISTRIBUTORS (P) LTD.

Management of Peripheral Nerve Injuries and Role of Tendon Transfer

Published by
Pawaninder P. Vij
Peepee Publishers and Distributors (P) Ltd.
160, Shakti Vihar, Pitam Pura
Delhi - 110034 (India)
Ph: 27020004, 9811156083
e-mail: peepee160@yahoo.co.in

First Edition: **2004**

ISBN 81-88867-03-9

Printed at
Lordson, C-5/19, Rana Pratap Bagh,
Delhi - 110 007.

Preface

Peripheral nerve injuries are common in day-to-day life activities, because these are superficially situated. Primarily general practitioners, surgeons or orthopedic surgeons deal these nerve injuries. When patient of nerve injuries report to plastic surgeon or the hand surgeon, situation is almost in irreversible state.

This book would be of use to trainee plastic surgeons AS well AS general surgeons and orthopedic surgeons. We have tried to give everything at one place.

I hope, readers would appreciate the efforts in taking out this small, concise but very useful book.

Vishwa Prakash

Contents

Chapter-1

Peripheral Nervous System

The nervous system is divided into two parts-central nervous system and peripheral nervous system. The central nervous system-the brain and its caudal prolongation the spinal cord, is connected to the periphery by the peripheral nervous system.

The peripheral nervous system includes the cranial nerves, the spinal nerves with their roots and rami, the peripheral nerves and the peripheral components of the autonomic nervous system.

The peripheral nerve

The peripheral nerves contain motor fibres (to end plates in the skeletal muscles), sensory fibres (from organs and endings in skin, muscle, tendon and joint), and autonomic fibres (to blood vessels, sweat glands and arrectores pilarium muscles).

The spinal nerves

These are thirty-one pairs of spinal nerves - eight cervical, twelve thoracic, five lumbar, five sacral and one coccygeal. All arise from the spinal cord. Each spinal nerve leaves or enters the cord by an anterior, largely motor root, and a posterior sensory root.

In adult the spinal cord extends caudally only so

far as the first lumbar vertebral level, the obliquity of the merging and entering roots in the theca increases from above downwards.

The lumbar and the sacral roots occupy the theca below the first lumbar level.

Anatomy of the peripheral nerves

A peripheral nerve is composed of the neuroepithelial conducting structures and the mesenchyme which supports and protects them. In a cross section examination the nerve appears in the form of several bundles held together by a mantle of connective tissue. These fibres are of two types-myelinated and non-myelinated.

Myelinated fibres

Each myelinated fibre is composed of the axon surrounded by a myelin sheath, the two elements being neatly enclosed in the Schwann cell.

The axon is the prolongation of the nerve cell and is surrounded by it's own membrane, known as axolemma.

The myelin sheath consists of lamellae arranged in regular spiral, which are formed from the cytoplasmic membrane of the Schwann cell.

Schwann cells are arranged in a chain, of which each link is approximately 1 millimeter long. A Ranvier's node is found between each two segments, in a short unsheathed area.

Sheaths of the nerve

The sheaths or the connective tissue is conveniently divided in three parts, the endoneurium, the perineurium and the epineurium.

The endoneurium comprises cells and an extra cellular ground substance. The cells are mainly fibroblasts and have no basement membrane.

The perineurium is the sheath containing one bundle inside.

The epineurium comprises all the connective tissue of nerve trunk out side the perineurium.

Blood supply of the nerves

Nerves have both an extrinsic and an intrinsic blood supply.

Extrinsic system of the blood supply consists of arteries and veins that accompany the nerve close to but not incorporated within the epineurium. This extrinsic system may accompany the nerve for a portion or all of its length. There are different patterns of relationships between the extrinsic system and the nerve.

1. No dominant extrinsic vessel supplying the nerve.
2. One dominant artery and the vein accompany the nerve for the majority of its length.
3. The nerve may be accompanied at different points by different dominant extrinsic systems.
4. The nerve may be supplied by one dominant longitudinal system that accompanies the nerve for part of its course but then departs leaving segments of the nerve without any dominant extrinsic system.
5. The blood supply to the nerve trunk may be from multiple dominant extrinsic vessels interspaced with free segments.

Intrinsic system consists of epineural, perineural, and endoneural vascular plexuses running longitudinally. There are extensive anastomoses between all of these systems. Under normal conditions, only part of the vessels is patent at any one time. Trauma may result in vasodilatation of the closed channels and even reversal of the flow.

Vasa nervosum is the connecting link between extrinsic and intrinsic system. These pass to the nerve through a sheet of thin areolar tissue referred to as the mesoneurium. These vessels are usually 3-5 cm apart, therefore a nerve can be stripped of its blood supply about 6-10 cm.

Chapter-2

What happens when a Nerve is Injured

The nerves can be damaged in a number of ways: ischemia;

- the effects of systemic disease;
- injuries-blunt, sharp cut, compression or stretch ing;
- infection and inflammatory processes.

Changes proximal to the lesion

The proximal to lesion, changes occur in the internal structure of the nerve cell. Within a few days there is a reduction in the caliber of proximal axon; there may be atrophy of whole axonal shaft. In the body there is chromatolysis and retraction of dendrites.

During the regenerative phase the proximal stump is the site of intense activity and multiplication of Schwann cells, migrating from proximal and distal stumps, forming the bands of Bunger.

The axons of the proximal stump sprout. Collateral sprouts arise from the nodes of Ranvier at levels at which the axons are still intact; terminal sprouts arise from the tip of the surviving axon.

With entry of axonal sprouts into the distal stump there is second wave of Schwann cell proliferation. Initially there are more axonal sprouts then there were axons in the intact nerve. But only those survive which establish the connection with end organs.

Initially the proximal stump becomes divided into mini fascicles, the arrangement is confined to the proximal stump and the gap; which is changed to usual arrangement of fibres after some months.

The gap between proximal and distal stump is first filled with blood containing macrophages: a fibrin clot is then formed. Into this clot proceed capillaries and fibroblasts from surrounding tissues and nerve ends.

The advancing axonal sprouts accompany Schwann cells. When the gap is bridged by the nerve graft, the latter acts as a source of the Schwann cells. The axons are able to traverse a 10-mm gap.

Changes distal to the lesion

Divided peripheral nerve undergoes secondary degeneration throughout its distal portion, which is separated from the trophic center. This is known as Wallerian degeneration. Axon and the myelin sheath is digested by the Schwann cell. It starts within 24 hours and reaches its peak in 7 days time. Whereas the axon and the myelin sheath are destroyed and disappear, the Schwann cell survives. It remains in a belt of cells known as Bugners band.

Evaluation of an acute traumatic peripheral nerve injury

At time of injury

Initially examination is done and diagnosis established. It works AS baseline against which progressive sensory or motor loss due to haemorrhage or edema is noted. Sensory and motor loss should be noted.

When a region traversed by a nerve is involved in

an open or closed injury, damage to the nerve should always be suspected until it can be excluded. The possibility of damage to a nerve at more than one level should be kept in mind where there are multiple wounds of the limb.

Diagnosis starts with careful history and the examination

History should include;

1. Onset and the course of the condition, and
2. The wounding mechanism including the site and the depth of a therapeutic injection, the use of tourniquet and legation of a vessel.

Examination includes: A systematically conducted clinical examination to reveal the status of motor, sensory and sympathetic functions.

If some time has elapsed since the injury and open wound has healed, the site of the injury should be palpated to ascertain if a neuroma is present on the nerve. Neuroma takes some time to develop and usually appear after 3 months of injury.

The percussion should be done to elicit Tinel's sign from below upwards. The presence of Tinel's sign is indication of regeneration.

Evaluation of the motor function should also be done.

1. The degree and distribution of muscle wasting should be noted.
2. The appearance or absence of visible palpable contractions in individual muscles in response to voluntary effort should be noted.
3. Measuremnet of range and power of individual

movements in response to voluntary effort should be noted.

Electrodiagnosis

A number of electro diagnostic methods are available for detecting the peripheral nerve injuries, for determining the level of lesion and for evaluating its severity, they include:

1. the muscle response to nerve trunk stimulation;
2. changes in the electrical excitability of the affected muscles;
3. the interpretation of muscle action potentials in EMG of the affected muscles;
4. changes in the conduction time and nerve conduction velocity of motor fibres AS determined by stimulation electromyography.

The manner in which the nerve functions are lost

1. Acute lesion
2. Chronic lesions

Acute lesions

This may date from injury or the nerve may be damaged during the procedures undertaken for the treatment of the injury such AS:

A. care less wound debridement or inadvertently clamping or ligating a nerve when controlling bleeding;

B. the reduction of fracture and dislocation;
C. the application of the tourniquet or ill fitting plaster;
D. a misplaced therapeutic injection;

In these cases the nerve may or may not have been left in continuity

Chronic lesions

These lesions are in continuity in which progressively increasing number of fibres are affected, individual fibres sustaining increasing damage AS the deforming force continues to operate. Such lesions may develop AS a result of:

1. complications introduced by an earlier injury; for example, injuries about the elbow joint AS in tardy ulnar palsy;
2. occupational compression;
3. entrapement neuropathies.

Nerve conduction block injuries

In these types of injuries, both continuity of the axon and overall microstructure of the nerve fibres are preserved.

Aetiology

Usually there are two reasons:

1. compression and,
2. ischemia.

Compression is divided into three groups:

a. transient conduction block which is of a few minutes or hour duration and, is without overt pathological changes and is primarily vascular in origin;

b. moderately severe lesion in which conduction block persists for unto 4 weeks. Pathological changes are then present in the injured segment, which is edematous, hyperemic, and infiltrated with macrophages and lymphocytes. There is thinning of axons, and myelin is granulated. Finally, thinned axons are left with only a thin coating of myelin;

c. the severe conduction block lesion in which the block persists for several months. Conspicuous pathological features were again axon thinning and segmental demyelination.

Role of ischemia

The structural integrity and the conduction properties depend upon a continuing and adequate blood supply. Compression ischemia, measured in minutes may block conduction.

The transition from a conduction block injury to onset of axonal degeneration is reached when ischemia is unrelieved for about 6 Hours.

If ischemia continues, conduction failure develops. If pressure is relieved circulation through the compressed segment improves and with this the changes are reversed and recovery follows. Failing this, the changes in the compressed segment proceed to the point where axons break down and Wallerian degeneration takes place.

Chapter-3

Role of Electromyography in Peripheral Nerve Injuries

An overall electromyogram with skin surface electrodes, ordinary electromyography, study of action potential after stimulations, and calculation of conduction velocities, provides the information, which makes it possible to refine the diagnosis.

Electromyograms following stimulation will enable detection of the first signs of reinnervation at a moment when the clinical tests are still negative. Subsequently, electromyography will make it possible to follow the development of the reinnervation.

EMG is of no value in open wound, but it is of value in closed wounds and in those wounds in which the nerve has ben repaired by somebody else.

In early stage, before Wallerian degeneration has taken place (21 days) and while electrical examination by stimulation still produces normal results, it will show the extent and distribution of neuronal deficiency.

Loss of motor units is shown AS

During effort by reduction in the number of motor unit potentials and an increase in their frequency to compensate for the dropping out of the paralyzed units.

Ar rest by spontaneous fibrillation.

When a nerve trunk is sectioned

Spontaneous fibrillatory activity consisting of small short lived potentials appears in the days following the accident. This change corresponds to spontaneous activity of muscle fibres, which has been isolated from neuronal control. It reached its peak, when Wallerian degeneration has become established and remains at that peak as long AS degeneration lasts.

If there is loss of conduction but no anatomical gap AS in compression

EMG pattern will be identical to that of nerve discontinuity. However it is relatively uncommon that there would not be few active motor units in such cases.

It can also help in deciding in the matters of nerve suturing whether to allow reinnervation or go for surgical revision.

Chapter-4
Nerve Suturing

Aims

The aim of the nerve repair is not only to restore continuity of the nerve trunk but to do so in a planned manner so that maximum functional recovery is achieved by:

1. maximizing the entry of axons into the distal stump, into fasciculi and into functionally related endoneurial tubes;
2. minimising the loss of regenerating axons into the interfascicular epineurial tissue of the distal stump;
3. restoring correct axial realignment of the nerve ends;
4. minimising the further retrograde loss of the neurons consequent on further trauma to the proximal nerve stump during its preparation for repair.

Microsurgery and the nerve repair

- Unaided eye has a limited place in the nerve surgery today.
- Microsurgery should be taken to mean surgery under magnification and not necessarily under operating microscope.
- Microsurgery has increased the accuracy of conventional epineurial repair by improving the correct alignment of the nerve ends and fascicular apposition. It provided a sharper definition of the

tissues at the nerve ends during their preparation for repair. It helps in using the ultrafine needles and suture materials. Postoperative fibrosis and neuroma formation at the suture site are reduced. Fascicular repair may also be done.

Freeing and mobilization of the nerve ends during repair

1. Nerve should not be approached directly through the scar tissue. It should always be identified and isolated well above and below.
2. Before disturbing the nerve, any visible landmark on the nerve surface, such AS arrangement of the blood vessels should be noted. This would assist in restoring correct alignment of the nerve ends when they are finally brought together.
3. The nerve ends from the surrounding scar tissues should be freed with care to avoid further trauma to the nerve, to avoid damage to intact branches in vicinity and, to preserve the blood supply to the nerve.

Preparation of the nerve ends

The particular attention should be given to following:

- to preserve the blood supply to the repair site.
- the nerve ends should be healthy;

The accepted practice is to trim the nerve ends carefully until the healthy bundles are exposed. It means that proximal face should present the fasciculi with well-defined outlines that glisten and pout somewhat from the nerve ends. Because the destruction of the fasciculi sometimes extends more irregularly along the nerve stumps, sectioning the nerve ends may expose some normal looking fasciculi before others. In these cases the trimming should be continued until conditions are equally favorable across the entire face of the nerve.

However it becomes very difficult to prepare the distal stumps. In delayed repair because the distinction between the fibrous tissue and fascicular tissue becomes less clear with atrophy of the latter tissue, so it is better to error on the more side than less.

Restoring correct alignment of the nerve ends

Restoration of the correct alignment is facilitated by:

1. use of identification markers prior to freeing the nerve or nerve ends from the scar tissue;
2. matching the blood vessles on the surface of the nerve;
3. matching the fasciculi at the nerve ends;
4. use of electrical and histochemical methods to identify fasciculi.

Repair

Diagrams showing different Nerve suturing methods:

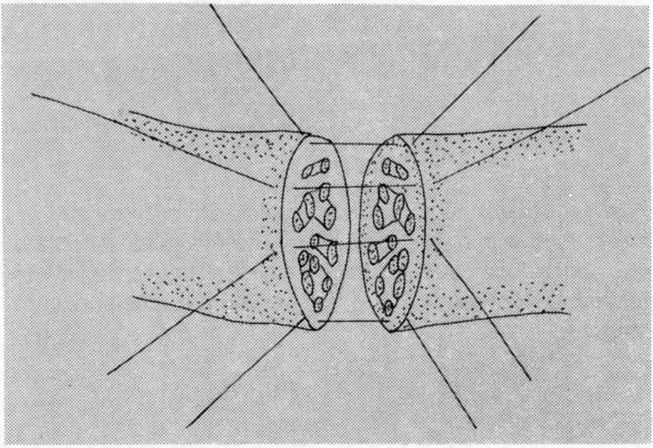

Fig. 4.1 Shows external epineurial repair, microsutures are placed in the epineurium adjacent to fascicles.

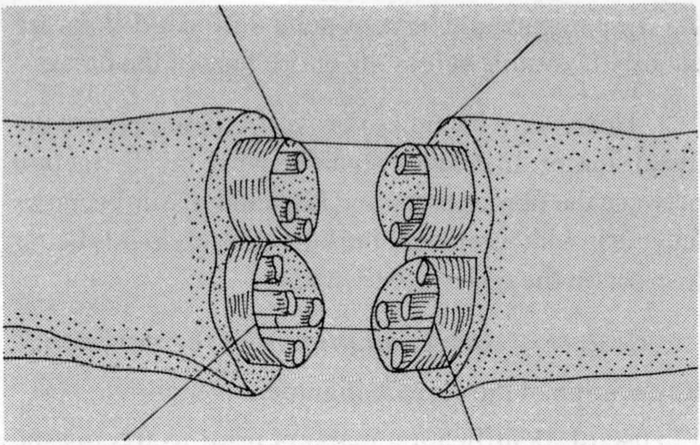

Fig. 4.2 Shows group fascicular repair, dominant groups of fascicles are separated and the perimeter of the groups sutured. Sutures are used to align the fascicles in each group.

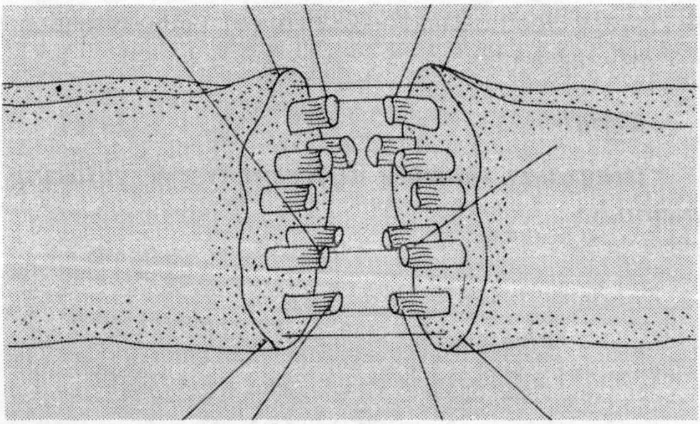

Fig. 4.3 Shows single fascicle repairs, two or three sutures are placed within the epineurium and the outer lamella of the perineurium to align each fascicle. This repair is very technically demanding and is reserved for special circumstances.

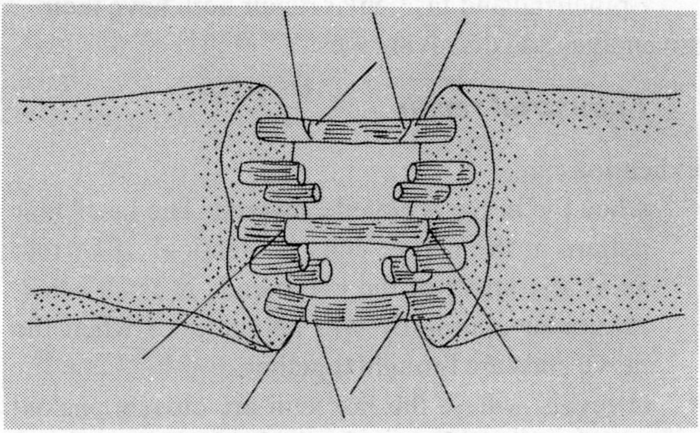

Fig. 4.4 Shows alignment of nerve grafts which is difficult because of dissimilar patterns of fascicle topography between nerve stumps and nerve graft.

End to end repair

Where the nerve ends may be brought together with out tension well executed epineural suture under magnification is best.

Few comments are:

- nerve suturing should be always performed under loupe magnification;
- suture material should be fine and non reactive;
- needle trauma should be minimum;
- sutures should be confined to superficial epineurium only, so that they , and the reaction they produce, are not in track of regenerating axons.
- function of the sutures is to hold the nerves together until healing is completed. So 2-6 sutures are adequate for most repairs;
- apposition should be loose and never tight. Tight union results in buckling of fascicular ends and force the cut ends of fasciculi into the inter fascicular tissues of both distal and proximal stumps.

Epineurial and fascicular repair both have their advantages and disadvantages

Epineurial repair

Indications are;

- when the nerve is cleanly severed .The fascicular pattern at the nerve ends is identical .If correct axial alignment of the nerve ends is established, fascicular continuity will be achieved when the nerve ends are brought together.
- at levels where the fasciculi are closely packed and there is little interfascicular epineurial tissue into which the regenerating axons can grow.

Group fascicular repair

Fascicular repair is misleading term giving the impression that the nerve is repaired fasciculus by fasciculus, on a one to one basis, so that fascicular continuity is restored in every aspect.

If we try to do one to one fascicular repair there would be suture line crowded with sutures aggravating the scar tissue formation.

Some of the fasciculi are so fine that to reunite them is very difficult.

In secondary repair, there would be difference of the size and it wont be possible to coapt one to one.

So Fascicular repair, essentially means group fascicular repair.

The aim of this is:

1. obtain the best possible fascicular apposition during the union so that regenerating axons are confined to fasciculi and, therefore, endonurial tubes;
2. reduce the chances of fasciculi becoming opposed to interfascicular tissue.

So correct axial alignment of the nerve ends is crucial

- where naturally occuring fascicular grouping can be identified at nerve ends this should be preserved;
- when there are no naturally occuring fascicular groupings, the fasciculi are then arranged arbitraily into groups in order to achieve the objectives listed above.

Group fascicular method is the best method in

1. Nerve grafting
2. When there is risk of sensory becoming opposed to motor fasciculi.

Tension free nerve union

1. Harden the nerve ends by freezing so that physical damage is minimized when they are being trimmed.

2. Use a sharp blade to trim the nerve ends and hold the nerve ends by wrapping in a sheath and applying the artery forceps.

Immediate repair should be carried out if possible. If it is not possible, two nerve ends should be brought together by means of two easily identified sutures so AS to avoid retraction.

In case of secondary surgery exploration of the one or more nerve trunks must proceed from the simple to the complex; uncovering the nerves above and below the lesions and a gradual dissection towards the scar area. There are two possibilities:

1. discontinuity of the nerve ends
2. nerve is in continuity.

Discontinuity of the nerve ends: If the nerve ends

are discontinuous, both ends are dissected. Most probably there would be terminal neuroma, which is excised till healthy looking axons appear. Most probably in such circumstances end to end suturing would be difficult unless the nerves were prevented to retract. If nerves can be brought together the suturing is done using one of the methods AS described. However if nerves can not be brought together, nerve grafting would be required.

If nerve is in continuity: If the nerve is in continuity there are two possibilities:

1. external compression;
2. internal damage.

For relieving external compression, neurolysis is done.

For internal damage internal neurolysis or intraneural dissection is done.

Neurolysis: Dissection is done longitudinally along the axis of the trunk, the bundles being freed from adherent scar above and below and also inside the nodule itself. The scar tissue is excised to healthy fibres and defect is replaced by the nerve graft.

Internal neurolysis is done under magnification. All the fibrous tissue is excised preserving the fibres in continuity. The defect so created is bridged by nerve grafts.

Chapter-5
Nerve Grafting

Indications

1. Large gaps.
2. Partial lesions-if exploration of the nerve shows lateral neuroma in relation to intact nerve fibres, damaged fibres are separated from intact nerve fibres. After resection of the neuroma the gap is neatly bridged by means of inlay graft.

Principles of nerve grafting

1. Cutaneous nerves are usually employed for grafting. The common donor in the upper limb is the medial cutaneous nerve of the forearm taken from the upper arm, in the lower limb, the sural nerve.
2. These cutaneous nerves have a cross - sectional diameter of 2-3 mm. and yield an average of 22-30 cm of the graft.
3. It some times happen that two main nerves are extensively damaged at the same time; in these circumstances part of the less important nerve may be used to graft its fellow.
4. Free nerve grafts are revascularized across their suture lines and also from the bed in which they lie. In early stages this latter means of the survival is probably the more important of the two. The metabolic requirements of a free graft in which the axons and myelin are still present were thought to

be higher than one in which these materials have been previously removed by phagocytosis. Therefore predegenerate graft is better.

5. Axon traverse the proximal suture line into the graft, the progress at the far end is barred by fibrous invasion of the distal suture line from the surrounding tissues. It is suggested that time taken for axons to traverse the graft should be calculated and at the time they were reckoned to have reached the distal suture line a resection and suture at this level should be undertaken.
6. The cross sectional area of the graft or grafts must be equal to that of the nerve to be repaired.
7. The graft should be longer than gap to be filled.
8. Bed should be free of scar tissue to facilitate revascularization.

Types of the grafts:

Inlay graft

Inlay nerve grafts are used in partial nerve injuries in which the lateral neuroma is formed. At operation damaged fibres are separated from the intact nerve fibres. After resection of the lateral neuroma the gap is bridged by strands of cutaneous nerve and secured by very fine sutures.

Cable graft

A cable graft is composed of several strands of a cutaneous nerve and is used to bridge a gap in the main trunk such AS median nerve in the forearm. The cross sectional diameter of the cable graft must, of course, be equal to that of the main trunk.

Pedicle graft

The principles of pedicle nerve grafting are similar to those that apply to grafting of the skin. At first stage the proximal neuroma of the both nerves are resected and the ends sutured together. The extent of the gap to be closed in the median nerve is noted. Ulnar nerve is then exposed in upper arm. And allowing for same shrinkage, the level at which the nerve must be divided is calculated.

The nerve is ligated at the level from which division is required later on.

The second stage is carried out not less than six weeks later.

The ulnar nerve is exposed again and divided in upper arm. It is mobilized to the point at which the nerves have been previously united.

The nerve graft is then passed subcutaneously in the forearm to the distal stump of the median nerve exposed at the wrist level. After resection of the stumps, the nerves are repaired in the usual way.

Tubal nerve repair

This involves the use of a vein, artery, mesothelial tube or a tube of some biodegradable material AS a conduit to facilitate the passage of regenerating axons across a nerve gap.

Predegenerate graft

Predegenerating graft by nerve section in situ 8-15 days before its removal improves regeneration and it is because:

1. such graft becomes firmer and are easy to handle.
2. axon and myelin sheath debris in degenerating nerve fibres in the graft obstruct the advance of axon and that, if sufficient time is allowed for endoneurial tubes to be cleared of this debris, regenerating axons will then advance more easily and rapidly.

3. increased metabolic activity associated with Wallerian degeneration and removal of debris would demand an increased blood supply. This is readily available when the graft is sectioned and left in situ. After fifteen days when the graft is transferred, endoneurial tubes will have cleared of debris, and graft would be able to withstand the initial and temporary reduction of loss of blood supply pending its revascularization.

Timing of the distal nerve graft repair

Normally the graft is attached proximally and distally at the same operation. However, there is always the risk that, by the time regenerating axons reach the distal suture line, scarring at that site will present an impenetrable barrier to their further advance. So distal end should be sutured later on, or excised and sutured later.

Direct neurotization of muscles

Neurotization is the direct implantation of the proximal stump of a transected nerve into a denervated muscle with the intention of reinnervating muscle fibres from the source. Though it has been described but reinnervation has not been proved clinically. Yes in some of following situations it can be used:

1. cross face reinnervation of the paralyzed muscles
2. when a branch or branches have been avulsed from the muscle.

Chapter-6

Indications and Timing of Secondary Repair

The usual fault with all surgeons is to wait too long before performing secondary repairs. AS a result, trophic movements, trick movements, muscular atrophy and joint changes start taking place; which are very difficult to correct.

Indication for secondary repair

Indications of secondary repair are never clear cut. There are different views. Author is of opinion that secondary repair should always be done because even if there is no or negligible possibility of motor recovery, nerve repair would at least achieve protective sensations.

Timing: Various authors have suggested different waiting time before secondary intervention. Lange waited 2 years, while on the other hand Deyerle and Tucker suggest performing tendon transfers at the same time AS the nerve repair.

Usual protocol

1. It is reasonable to wait for about 4 months.

If no sign of recovery:

Explore the nerve.

If nerve repair is of good quality: do interfascicular neurolysis.

If nerve repair is poor: again repair preferably with a graft.

2. If 4 months after the primary repair, there are signs of recovery of sensations,

- Wait longer
- But if after 6 months and repeated EMG studies no sign of motor recovery, exploration of the nerve is again indicated.

3. If there is proximal motor recovery, but opposition is not recovered , don't wait for more than 9 months. Same is true for proximal ulnar nerve repair. Recovery of intrinsic muscles is poor. So it is advisable to consider palliative procedures.

- However, in radial nerve lesions, recovery is very frequent because of proximal situations of muscles supplied by the radial nerve .In division of the radial nerve at the mid humerus, transfer should be delayed 6 months or longer after neurorrhaphy.

What author recommends?

Author recommends immediate tendon transfer in all patients

Reasons

After nerve repair regeneration of the nerve takes long time. During which massage of the joints and the stimulation of the muscles is mandatory along with various splints. In our country patients' compliance for above mentioned procedures is very poor because of various factors. Author has come across many patients in whom sensory recovery was excellent but motor improvement was not present, because till nerve regeneration took place, joint contractures have developed and the motor end plates have degenerated. Therefore considering all the factors; author is doing primary tendon transfer in all the patients with good results .If the patient has come after the nerve repair done somewhere else, author does tendon transfer whenever patient presents.

Chapter-7

How to Improve the Results of Nerve Repair

There are few of the factors, which, if taken in account can improve the results of the nerve repair, such AS:

1. prevention and treatment of wound infection
2. the introduction of the microsurgical techniques
3. avoid the rough technique while preparing the proximal end
4. to prevent suture line scarring to minimum. Suture line scarring impairs axonal regeneration by obstructing the advance of some regenerating axons, constricting regenerating axons, thereby slowing their progress, impairing the blood supply of the region.

The suture line scarring can be minimized by:

a. avoiding tension at suture line
b. taking care that blood supply at suture line is adequate and not damaged, which can be achieved by:
    1. When mobilizing the nerves extrinsic longitudinal arterial anastomotic system should be avoided.

2. The most favourable and well vascularized bed should be found for nerve repair, even if this means rerouting the nerve.
3. Wrapping the suture site should be avoided, AS it inhibits the revascularization of suture area from the nerve bed.
4. Major vessels severed by the injury should be avoided.
5. Every effort should be made to limit the fibrosis at suture line.
6. If autograft is used, use vascularized graft, and avoid graft of large fascicles AS there is risk of central necrosis.

Measures to promote entry of regenerating axons in the distal stump

a. Immeditae repair of nerve.
b. Obtain correct axial alignment and match related fascicular group by matching blood vessels on the surface of the nerve.
c. Careful inspection of the nerve ends may reveal some distinctive fasciculi that have retained there identity at each nerve end.
d. Electrical stimutaion of fasciculi at the nerve ends in order to identify motor and sensory fasciculi.
   At distal nerve ends
   Failure to elicit a motor response is accepted AS evidence that it is sensory fasciculus.
   At proximal end
   In proximal end stimulation would elicit patients reaction if the sensory fasciculus is there.

Measures for peripheral tissues

The denervated peripheral tissues should be preserved in best possible condition pending their reinnervation.

Chapter-8

Sural Nerve and Vascularized Sural Nerve Graft

Sural nerve is most commonly used nerve AS the graft

Anatomy

- Branch of tibial nerve.
- Descends between the heads of Gastrocnemius muscle.
- Pierces deep fascia proximally in leg and joined by sural communicating branch of common peroneal.
- Descends lateral to tendocalcaneus to the region between lateral malleolus and the calcaneum.
- Proceeding distal to the lateral malleolus along the latreal side of foot and little toe.
- It is long 35-40 cm with a well-recognized intramural fascicular structure.

Blood supply

- Superficial sural artery derived either directly from the popliteal artery, or else from sural artery. It gives off several cutaneous branches and follow the nerve almost along its entire length, usually ending in lower third of the leg by anastomosing with an ascending branch of posterior tibial artery.

- The artery supplies the nerve with an average of seven nutrient arteries, with a gap of 4-6 cm between each

Surgical approach

- Prone position.
- Longitudinal posterior incision in the leg.
- In popliteal fossa the vascular pedicle is easily identified and followed to its origin.
- Nerve is removed en block with its perineurial structures consisting of the artery and the vein.
- The nerve is detached at both the ends and at release of tourniquet, the blood supply can be checked.
- If the loss of substance is fairly short and several strands are needed, dividing the intraneural constituents while maintaining the vascular pedicle intact can preserve the blood supply.

Indications of vascualrized nerve grafts

1. Tissue loss in unfavourable bed.
2. Use of large nerve trunks in very extensive lesions.

Physiotherapy and functional rehabilitaion after the lesions of the the peripheral nerves

Physical treatment and functional reeducation are required only in cases of axontmesis and neurotmesis. In neuropraxia, axons remain intact and there is only short lived interruption of the nerve conduction. Loss of sensory and motor function in neuropraxia is usually restored in few weeks time.

A closed injury and the injuries in which the nerves are repaired by somebody else

Most of the time even with refined electrodiagnostic examination, it is difficult to differentiate between axontmesis and neurotmesis. Indeed, in axontmesis and neurotmesis, the initial clinical and electrical signs are identical.

Whether neurotmesis (When nerve has been repaired) or axontmesis, regeneration of the axons and the myelin sheath will require considerable time, the length of which depends to a greater extent on the latent period before the process begins (About thirty days):

- distance between site of the lesion and the muscles dependent on the part of the nerve which has been damaged (The average speed of regeneration of the nerve fibre is roughly 1 mm per day), and
- in the case of suture the time which elapses between the injury and the surgical procedures.

Aim

Aim of physiotherapy and functional rehabilitation after lesions of the peripheral nerve are:

- to prevent contracture formation;
- to keep the joints soft and supple;
- to prevent disuse atrophy of muscles;
- to prevent damage to the skin;
- to prevent contracture formation.

Causes

1. Disturbed balance between certain group of muscles (agonists and antagonists), like adduction contracture of the thumb in median nerve palsy.
2. Musculotendinous or aponeurotic retractions.
3. The reaction of adhesions between various layers of tissues.
4. Periarticular or articular stiffness.

For example, there would be no point in having successfully sutured a radial nerve, if by the time recovery takes place, there is irreducible deformity, AS stiffness of wrist.

How to prevent

1. Physiotherapy
2. Splinatge

To prevent atrophy of muscles: Any muscle completely and permanently deprived of its innervation will undergo metabolic disturbances and histological changes which will finally lead to total disappearance of its fibres and their replacement by functionless fibroadipose tissue.

Studies have shown that if reinnervation occurs within one year, satisfactory recovery can be anticipated. On the other hand, after three years, there is no justification for expecting a positive result unless it has been possible to slow up the process of muscle atrophy and degeneration.

Causes of atrophy

AS early AS three days after section of the nerve, there is onset of atrophy, which will reach a peak at the end of 40 days and will involve an average loss of 75% of the original weight of the healthy muscle. Causes are:

1. lack of neurotrophic influence exerted by normal axons on muscle fibres
2. disorders of blood and lymph capillaries of muscle itself
3. complex metabolic disturbances probably of enzymatic origin and the regulation of which is said to depend on the intactness of the axons

4. excessive fatigue resulting from fibrillation, immobilization, and finally temperature; since exposure to cold accelerates rate of atrophy.

How to prevent

1. Local application of the heat
2. Massage
3. Electrical stimulation by the galvanic current.

Chapter-9

Physiotherapy and Functional Rehabilitaion after the Lesions of the Peripheral Nerves

Physical treatment and functional re-education are required only in cases of axontmesis and neurotmesis. In neuropraxia, axons remain intact and there is only short lived interruption of the nerve conduction. Loss of sensory and motor function in neuropraxia is usually restored in few weeks time.

A closed injury and the injuries in which the nerves are repaired by somebody else

Most of the time even with refined electrodiagnostic examination, it is difficult to differentiate between axontmesis and neurotmesis. Indeed, in axontmesis and neurotmesis, the initial clinical and electrical signs are identical.

Whether neurotmesis (When nerve has been repaired) or axontmesis, regeneration of the axons and the myelin sheath will require considerable time, the length of which depends to a greater extent on the latent period before the process begins (About thirty days):

- distance between site of the lesion and the muscles dependent on the part of the nerve which has been damaged (The average speed of regeneration of the nerve fibre is roughly 1 mm per day), and:
- in the case of suture the time which elapses between the injury and the surgical procedures.

Aim

Aim of physiotherapy and functional rehabilitation after lesions of the peripheral nerve are:

- to prevent contracture formation;
- to keep the joints soft and supple;
- to prevent disuse atrophy of muscles;
- to prevent damage to the skin;
- to prevent contracture formation .

Causes

1. Disturbed balance between certain group of muscles (agonists and antagonists), like adduction contracture of the thumb in median nerve palsy.
2. Musculotendinous or aponeurotic retractions.
3. The reaction of adhesions between various layers of tissues.
4. Periarticular or articular stiffness.

For example, there would be no point in having successfully sutured a radial nerve, if by the time recovery takes place, there is irreducible deformity, AS stiffness of wrist.

How to prevent

1. Physiotherapy
2. Splinatge

To prevent atrophy of muscles: Any muscle completely and permanently deprived of its innervation will undergo metabolic disturbances and histological changes which will finally lead to total disappearance of its fibres and their replacement by functionless fibroadipose tissue.

Studies have shown that if reinnervation occurs within one year, satisfactory recovery can be anticipated. On the other hand, after three years, there is no justification for expecting a positive result unless it has been possible to slow up the process of muscle atrophy and degeneration.

Causes of atrophy

AS early AS three days after section of the nerve, there is onset of atrophy, which will reach a peak at the end of 40 days and will involve an average loss of 75% of the original weight of the healthy muscle. Causes are:

1. lack of neurotrophic influence exerted by normal axons on muscle fibres;
2. disorders of blood and lymph capillaries of muscle itself;
3. complex metabolic disturbances probably of enzymatic origin and the regulation of which is said to depend on the intactness of the axons;
4. excessive fatigue resulting from fibrillation, immobilization, and finally temperature; since exposure to cold accelerates rate of atrophy.

How to prevent

1. Local application of the heat.
2. Massage.
3. Electrical stimulation by the galvanic current.

Chapter-10

Ischaemic Nerve Lesions due to Trauma

Some facts about ischaemic nerve lesions are:

- adequate blood supply is essential for proper functioning of the nerve;
- if a nerve is deprived of its blood supply, it may receive oxygen by diffusion from the adjacent vascularized tissue, however it is true for smaller nerves only;
- when the blood supply of the nerve is impaired, nerve conduction is lost before the nerve suffers any structural damage. With increasing and continued ischemia, Wallerian degeneration occurs and nerve is finally converted into the fibrous cord;
- ischemia may be due to blockage of vessels or due to compression;
- critical time when ischemic lesion is converted into irreversible is 4-8 hours. At this time endoneurial edema appears which reflects damage to capillaries.

Classification

Nerve lesions due to ischemia may be classified AS,

1. Non-traumatic in origin

- due to arterial embolism,

- due to narrowing and occlusion of the arteria nervorum,
- arterial spasm and pathology from injection of harmful substances.

2. Traumatic in origin

- Indirect interference with blood supply AS in compression and stretch.
- Damage to arteria nervorum.
- Damage to main artery of the limb.
- Combined neurovascular injury.

Ischemic lesions are divided into four grades
Grade one and two:

Acute ischemia leads to a first and second degree injury, depending upon how quickly an collateral circulation develops. If circulation is restored rapidly there may be no Wallerian degeneration.

- If the restoration of the circulation is delayed, ischemia leads to Wallerian degeneration. If local circulation is restored before more advanced structural changes develop, the preserved endoneurial tubes, transmit regenerating axons to the periphery in such a way that function is fully restored.

Grade three: Chronic or prolonged ischemia is followed by more severe and permanent destruction of the nerve tissues. In a well established lesion, a considerable length of the nerve is affected; this is thinned, fibrotic and firm to palpation.

Grade 4 lesions: In these lesions the nerve is converted into a relatively avascular grossly shrunken, fibrotic strand, which may loose its identity in the scar tissues.

Management

1. The aetiological factor should be removed.
2. Nerve should be explored.
3. Under magnification damage should be assesed, and internal or combined neurolysis should be done.
4. In extensive damage, the involved segment may need removal and replacement with nerve graft.

Chapter-11

Nerve Injuries caused by Injection of the Therapeutic Agents

These nerve injuries are caused by therapeutic agent, which is inadvertently injected directly into the nerve or into the tissues immediatley surrounding it.

Nerve may be damaged by:

1. the needle AS it passes into or through the nerve is such a way that it penetrate the fasciculi;
2. toxic action of the agent;
3. the injection of the material into the fasciculus, which damages some of the nerve fibres and compresses others;
4. the injection of the material into the interfascicular tissues. The fibrosis, which follows constricts the fasciculi and impairs their blood supply;
5. direct injection into a major nutrient vessel;
6. involvement of nutrient vessles causing spasm or thrombosis, followed by the ischemic necrosis of nerve tissues.

Injection injuries may be localized to a few fasciculi or have wide spread effect depending on the way in which the lesion is produced. Intraneural injections are more damaging than extraneural and the consequences are far more serious.

Pathological findings may be:

1. intense inflammation and early fibrotic reaction about the nerve, which may appear swollen;
2. late findings may include thickened and shrunken nerve, may show a lateral neuroma, paraneural scarring with dense adhesions firmly binding the nerve to surrounding tissues, and intraneural fibrosis, confirmed by internal neurolysis;
3. lesions are usually localized.

Presentation

- In most case the onset is immediate or follows within a few minutes.
- A delayed onset suggests a more slowly acting agent and its location in the surrounding tissues.
- There is intense pain, which usually persists.
- Severe pain is the most disturbing feature of the lesion, taking on the characteristic of causalgia and finally requiring sympathetic block.

Management

Indications for exploration

1. The injection agent is known to be particularly toxic.
2. Severe persistent pain.
3. If after six weeks the recovery is not of acceptable standard.

Objections to early exploration

1. Some patients will recover in due course of time.
2. Unnecessary operative manipulations may add to the damage to the nerve.
3. Exploration does not always remove the difficulty of deciding in doubtful case, whether or not to

excise the damaged segment and repair the nerve.

Usually one should wait for 6 weeks so that any spontaneous recovery from a reversible conduction block lesion can be given a reasonable opportunity to reveal itself.

Exploration at or after 6 weeks is justified because

1. In experienced hand operation presents no problem.
2. State of the nerve may be confirmed.
3. Severe damage in the form of extensive necrosis may be identified and some form of surgical repair may be carried out.
4. Constrictive scars may be removed by internal and external neurolysis.

Chapter-12

Neuromas

An important function of the Schwann cells and endo neurial sheath is to insulate axons from the surrounding tissues. If this limiting barrier is destroyed, regenerating axons escape into, and branch freely within, a disorganized mass of fibrobalsts and Schwann cells to form a swelling, known AS neuroma.

The development, structure and size of neuroma depend on the number of axons that emerge from ruptured endoneurial tubes into surrounding tissues.

Neuromas may be:

1. neuromas in nerve in continuity;
2. terminal neuromas
3. suture line neuromas
4. amputation stump neuromas.

Neuromas on nerves in continuity

Neuromas on nerves in continuity are of two main types:

1. those in which perineurial sheath is not broken;
2. those in which the perineurial sheath is broken.

Lesions in which the perineurium is not broken (Pseudoneuromas)

Spindle shaped swellings may develop on the nerves where they are subjected to repeated friction or irritation.

- Initially the enlargement is due to an increase in connective tissue of the nerve, nerve fibres escaping direct injury.
- If irritation continues, nerve fibres suffer both from direct injury and indirectly from the deepening fibrosis that constricts the nerve fibres and impair their blood supply.

Symptoms

- paresthesia
- deepening numbness of the area served by the affected nerve
- severe pain when the swelling is compressed or the nerve is stretched.

Example

Bowlers thumb-in which the medial digital nerve is repeatedly compressed AS the thumb is firmly held against the edge of the ball.

Neuroma formation when the perineurium is ruptured by the injury

When some fasciculi are breached or severed, regenerating axons escape into interfascicular epineurial tissue where they continue to grow, branch and ramify widely in a disorganized way.

Suture line neuroma

There is high incidence of neuroma formation at the site of nerve repair. Where there are marked dissimilarities in the fascicular pattern at the nerve ends, cut ends of some fasciculi in the proximal stump will become opposed to interfascicular tissues on the distal stump during the repair. Consequently when the axons regenerate, large numbers of the axons enter interfascicular epineurial tissue forming a neuroma.

A large tender suture line neuroma developing in this way is an indication of the failed repair.

Treatment

1. Protect the neuroma from compression and traction.
2. Assess the nerve regeneration .If the recovery is not acceptable, go for excision and repair. However if recovery is acceptable, one can observe.

Amputaion stump neuromas

Following the amputation of a limb, neuromas form at the ends of the divided nerves. These neuromas present all the features of neuromas forming on the proximal stumps of a severed nerve. These are subjected to repeated blows, pressure and irritation.

Treatment

1. Transplantation of the cut ends into soft tissues AS muscles. Here axonal growth is deregulated, regenerating axons become widely dispersed and lost in tissues instead of attempting to confine and concentrate then at nerve ends. This is axonal deregulation.
2. Axonal regulation is also done, in which the nerve is pulled down, cleanly cut shortened, and after treating and capping the nerve ends, allowing it to retract into a pressure free bed. Simple ligation at two levels, 1. cm apart, combined with the use of chemical coagulant before finally enclosing the stump in a silastic cap is another alternative
3. Cross uniting the stumps of two nerves.

Non-operative methods

1. Desensitization.
2. Steroid injections.

Desensitization

Repeated nerve stimulation, percussion, massage, and ultrasound; all have been recommended. These work by blocking the painful stimuli, suppression of abnormal neurons, and induction of fibrous reaction, which protects the nerve endings.

However it is effective only during first three months after injury.

Steroid injection

Injection of triamcinolon (.2 to 1 ml) was given directly. This works by directly stabilizing the cell membrane and reducing the action potential instead of working AS an anti-inflammatory agent.

Chapter-13

Non-surgical Management of Pain Secondary to Peripheral Nerve Injuries

Pain after peripheral nerve injuries is quite common. AS a result of peripheral nerve injury, areas for spontaneous neural discharge are frequently established. These can take the form of neuroma or ectopic foci along the nerve. Leakage of norepinephrine from damaged sympathetic nerve fibres can result in abnormal sensitivity to normal stimuli. Spontaneous discharge from dorsal root ganglion and probably other CNS areas further complicates neurotransmission or pain perception.

Treatment

Acut phase of pain

Narcotic analgesics combined with non-narcotic analgesics with firm assurance.

Chronic persistent pain

The definition of the word chronic is almost totally arbitrary when defining pain. Any pain persisting beyond 3 weeks of nerve injuries or appearing after pain free interval is termed chronic pain. Causes of chronic pain are:

- scar tissue formation;
- neuroma formation ;
- symapathetic dystrophy (Overactivity);
- adeafferentation state producing central pain syndrome.

Management

Medical

1. Use of narcotics-best avoided.
2. Nonsteroidal anti-inflammatory drugs - Good.
3. Calcium channel blocking drugs and vasodilating drugs:

- Phenoxybenzamine is good and to be used in starting doses of 10 mg t.i.d., increasing gradually over several days to 60-80 mg per day;
- Nifedipine is another best drug in doses of 10mg t.i.d.;

4. Psychotropic drugs and related agents:

- tricyclic antidepressants -doses of 25-50 mg of amitryptiline may be effective;
- carbamazapine (Tegretol) is an anticonvulasant drug that may prove useful in central pain states. An adequate trial in each patient with doses from 1400-1600 mg per day are required for a period of six weeks prior to discontinuing the drug.

Therapeutic nerve blocks

1. Local infiltration or conduction block.
2. Regional sympathetic ganglion block.
3. Epidural block (Intermittent or continuous)

4. Intravascular regional techniques.
5. Neurolytic nerve blocks.

Electrical stimulation techniques

Surgically implantable electrical stimulation techniques have been found to be of use for pain relief.

Other peripheral stimulating techniques such AS use of TENS (transcutaneous electrical nerve stimulation) had been found to be effective by inhibition of spinothalamic tract cells and release of spinal cord endorphins.

Chapter-14

Individual Nerves and Common Tendon Transfers

Facial nerve

Anatomy

- Has a motor and a sensory root.
- The two roots emerge at the caudal border of pons.
- Pass anterolaterally with vestibulo cochlear nerve to internal acoustic meatus.
- Then descends to stylomastoid foramina.
- Emerging from stylomastoid foramina, the nerve runs forwards in the parotid gland, deep to the styloid process, retromanbdibular vein and external carotid artery and divides behind the neck of mandible into branches which pierce the anterolateratl surface of the parotid gland.

Then the nerve is divided into many branches to supply the facial muscles.

Branches

In facial canal

Nerve to stapedius
Chorda tympani

At exit from stylomastoid foramina

- Muscular branches to supply posterior auricular,

digastric posterior belly and,stylohyoid

On face

Five branches:

Temporal, zygomatic, buccal, marginal mandibular, and cervical.

Types of injuries

1. Acute Injuries and Bells palsy.
2. Chronic.

Management

1. *Aute injuries*

   Explore the wound and try to do end to end anastomosis.

2. *Acute infections*

   Medical treatment for 3-6 months.

   If no response-Neurolysis.

   If no response after neurolysis, and 6 months have passed it should be treated by various available methods like nerve transfer etc.

3. *Chronic*

- Tumors
- Chronic infections AS in leprosy.

In establishes paralysis

1. Less than 2 years duration

   Cross facial nerve grafting

2. More than 2 years duration

1. Muscle transfers (Dynamic Transfers)

- temporalis
- masseter

2. Static

- fascia lata sling

3. Staic on dynamic transfers (Authors technique)
4. Cross face nerve grafting with microneuro muscle transfer.

Though there are various methods available for treatment of facial palsies, author thinks that temporalis transfer is the best available option with internal splinting (Static on dynamic transfer).

Temporalis transfer

Muscle

- Arises like a fan from most of the temporal fossa, and from the deep surface of the temporal fascia.
- Its fibres converge and descend into a tendon that passes between the zygomatic arch and cranial wall and is inserted to medial surface, apex, anterior and posterior border of the coronoid process, and anterior border of the mandibular ramus almost to the third molar.

Nerve supply

Deep temporal; branches of mandibular nerve, passing above the lateral pterygoid to enter the deep surface of the temporalis. These are accompanied by deep temporal arteries.

Incision

Curved incision, which is an upward extension of preauricular incision.

Three smaller incisions, one at nasolabial grroove, and two at upper and lower lips just beyond midline on healthy side.

One small incision at medial canthus

At times one incision is also required at lateral canthus.

Procedure

- Temporalis fascia is exposed
- Five slips are made
- Slips are detached from inferior end while kept attached at upper end along with periosteum with temporalis muscle.
- Five slips of temporalis muscle are also made.
- Musculoaponeurotic slings are turned down and inserted to dermis through five incisions.
- Cross over is to be achieved at angle of mouth by passing the anterior slip to lower lip and posterior slip to upper lip.
- The slings are tied in tension
- Dressing done

Static support

This is done only for correction of the angle of the mouth.

Fascia lata is used

Three slings are made

One sling is attached to nasolabial fold and two others are attached to upper and lower lips.

The distal end is attached to zygomatic arch.

Author's technique

Author has recommended simultaneous static support AS well AS dynamic muscle transfer. This is due to fact that after muscle transfer splinting is essential. However in facial palsy the external splinting is not effective, and at times the muscle is strecthed. Stretched muscle loses its function. So Static support would basically act AS internal splint.

Chapter-15
Radial Nerve

Anatomy

- Arises from posterior cord C5, 6, 7, 8, T1.
- Descends behind third part of axillary artery.
- With the arteria profunda brachii and later, its radial collateral branch, it inclines dorsally.
- Then it passes obliquely across the back of the humerus first between the lateral and medial heads of the triceps, then in a shallow groove deep to the lateral head.
- On reaching the lateral side of the humerus it pierces the lateral inter muscular septa to enter the anterior compartment.
- Then it descends in a furrow between brachialis and brachioradialis proximally, and brachialis and extensor carpi radialis longus distally.
- Anterior to the lateral epicondyle it divides into superficial and deep terminal rami.

Branches

Muscular: To triceps, anconeus, brachioradialis, extensor carpi radialis longus and brachialis

Cutaneous: Posterior cutaneous nerve of the arm, lower lateral cutaneous nerve of the arm and, posterior cutaneous nerve of the forearm

Superficial terminal branch

- Descends from lateral epicondyle anterolaterally

in proximal 2/3 of forearm.

- At first on supinator, lateral to radial artery and behind the brachioradialis.
- In the middle third it is behind brachioradialis, close to lateral side of the radial artery.
- It leaves the artery 7 cm proximal to the wrist.
- Pierces the deep fascia and divides into 4-5 digital nerves.
- Digital nerves supply radial side of the thumb, first web space and second and third fingers upto IP joint.

Deep terminal branch

- Also known AS posterior interosseous nerve.
- Reaches the back of forearm round the lateral aspect of the radius between two sets of the fibres of supinator.
- Supplies all extensor muscles of forearm. Lie at first between superficial and deep extensor muscles, then passes deep to EPL and diminished to a thread upto dorsum of wrist ending AS a pseudo ganglion.

How to manage

Motor:

Usually there is wrist drop due to radial nerve injury. However triceps may also be involved if the injury is higher up. And in such cases extension of elbow is also impaired.

Sensory

Usually not much. However, injury causes loss of sensation over first web space.

Motor.

After injury all precautions should be taken to prevent atrophy and joint contracture by massage and galvanic stimulation. Cock up splint keeps the wrist in dorsiflexed position and avoids the wrist joint contracture .

Usually internal splinting by using pronator teres has been described in the books, author advises for triple transfer in acute cases of neurotmesis.

Management of nerve injury is same AS described before.

Triple transfer

Triple transfer is the basis of muscle transfer because in radial nerve palsy usually three functions are to be restored.

1. Extension of the wrist.
2. Extension of the thumb.
3. Extension of fingers at MP Joints.

Extension of the wrist

Usual muscle to be transferred is Pronator teres.

Extension of the thumb

Usual muscle to be transferred is Palmaris longus.

Extension of fingers

Usual muscle to be transferred is Flexor carpi ulnaris

How to transfer

Incision

- **On the flexor** aspect of forearm.
- A long curvilinear incision extending from pisiform proximally to the junction of uppermost and middle third of the forearm.
- **On dorsal** aspect of forearm.
- An L shaped incision, the transverse component of which lies at the level of the proximal border of extensor retinacula.

Identification of the tendons

- Through the dorsal incision a rectangular window is cut in deep fascia , so that all the extensor tendons are opened.
- The extensor digitorum and extensor pollicis longus are isolated and picked up by guide sutures.
- The tendon of abductor pollicis longus is also identified and picked up with a guide suture.
- Through the anterior incision, flexor carpi ulnaris is divided at its insertion and freed by sharp dissection from its origin from ulna.
- Through same incision palmaris logus is also mobilized.
- At upper border pronator teres is isolated.
- All the three tendons are transferred posteriorly.
- Pronator teres is transferred to ECRB.
- Palmaris longus is transferred to Extensor pollicis longus.
- Flexor carpi ulnaris is transferred to Extensor digitorum.

Authors modification

Author recommends taking flexor carpi radialis instead of ulnaris. He advises taking one half of ulnaris and transfer that to insertion of FCR. FCR is transferred to Ext.digitorum.

Postoperatively wrist is splinted in dorsiflexion and thumb in extension Fingers are splinted in slight flexion so AS to avoid the shortening of collateral ligament.

Chapter-16
Ulnar Nerve

Anatomy

- Arises from the medial cord.
- Runs distally through axilla, medial to axillary artery and between it and the vein.
- Continues distally medial to brachial artery AS far AS mid arm, here it pierces the medial intermuscular septum.
- Descends to the interval between medial epicondyle and the olecranon, with superior ulnar collateral artery.
- At elbow it lies in a groove on dorsum of epicondyle.
- It enters the forearm between two heads of flexor carpi ulnaris.
- Descends to the medial side of forearm on FDP, covered proximally by the flexor carpi ulnaris, its lower half covered by skin and fascia, is lateral to this muscle.
- In upper third of forearm, it is distant from ulnar artery but distal to this is close to its medial side.
- About 5 cm proximal to wrist it gives off dorsal branch, which continues distally in the hand, anterior to flexor retinaculum distal to pisiform bone.
- It passes behind the superficial part of the flexor retinacula with artery and divides into superficial and deep terminal branches.

Branches

Muscular

FCU and medial half of FDP.

Palmar cutaneous branch

Dorsal branch

Arises 5 cm proximally to wrist, passes distally and backwards, deep to FCU, perforates the deep fascia and divides into the digital nerves.

Superficial terminal branch

Supplies palmaris brevis and medial palmar skin and divides into two palmar digital nerves, which supply ulnar side of little finger and adjacent sides of little and ring fingers.

Deep terminal branch

- Deep terminal branch passes with deep branch of the ulnar artery, passes between the abductor digiti minimi and flexpr digiti minimi.
- And then follows deep palmar arch dorsal to flexor tendons.
- At its origin it supplies three hypothenar muscles,
- Then it supplies all interossei, 3rd and 4th lumbricals and ends by supplying the adductor pollicis.

How to manage

Motor: here is paralysis of FCU and half of FDP all interossei, ulnar two lumbricals and adductor pollicis.AS a result there is claw hand and loss of key pinch.

Sensory

There is loss of sensations in medial one and half of fingers on palmar aspect and medial two and half fingers on dorsal aspect.

What is claw hand.

Claw hand results due to paralysis of interrossei and lumbrical muscles which are prime flexors of MP joints and extensor of IP joints. When MP flexion is lost, there is hyperextension at MP joints due to unopposed action of Extensor digitorum, AS a result fingers at PIP joints undergo in flexion due to tenodesis effect.

Problem: Patient is not able to grasp properly. For proper grasp, first there should be MP flexion followed by IP flexion. In Claw hand MP flexion is not possible, instead there is flexion of IP joints followed by MP flexion due to long flexors and so grasp is not possible.

Management

Management is same as for other nerve injuries. The splint prescribed for such patients is known AS lumbrical splint in which the MP joints are kept in flexion.

Operative procedures

1. Dynamic transfers
2. Adynamic transfers

Tendon transfer

1. For Claw hand, there are various tendons available, however the most commonly used tendon is ECRB. It is used AS 4 tail procedure.

2. For loss of key pinch and loss of adductor function the FDS is used.

ECRB 4 tail transfer

Incisions

1. On dorsum of hand and forearm:

- small transverse incision at few mm beyond wrist;
- further two or three incisions on forearm .

2. On fingers:

- on medial side of index fingers;
- on lateral side of other fingers.

Procedure

- ECRB is detached from insertion.
- It is exposed in forearm and pulled back.
- Fascia lata is taken and anastomosed to ECRB.
- Four slips are made.
- Slips are taken in finger incisons by tendon tunneler. For this first the tendon tunneler is inserted from the incison in fingers, which passes palmar to deep transverse ligament and then passes dorsally to bring the slips of fascia in the finger incisions.

How to adjust the tension

- First slip to index finger is stitched.
- Then slip to little finer is stitched with tension that when it is pulled the index finer moves.
- Other two slips are stitched in moderate tension.
- POP is applied with wrist in dorsiflexion and fingers in MP flexion and IP extension

Adynamic procedures are used when dynamic procedure can not be used

Dermodesis

In this adynamic procedure the MP flexion is achieved by excising the skin and creating a contracture like state at MP joints.

Chapter-17

Medial Nerve

Anatomy

- Arises from two roots from lateral and medial cord of brachial plexus.
- Embrace the third part of axillary artery, uniting either anterior or lateral to it.
- Enters the arm at first lateral to the brachial artery, near the insertion of coracobrachialis it crosses in front of artery, descending medial to it to the cubital fossa; where it is posterior to bicipital aponeurosis and anterior to brachialis.
- Enters the forearm between the heads of pronator teres, crossing to the lateral side of the ulnar artery.
- Proceeds behind a tendinous bridge between humero-ulnar and radial heads of FDS, descending posterior and adherent to FDS and anterior to FDP.
- About 5 cm proximal to flexor retinaculum it emerges from behind the lateral edge of FDS, becoming superficial just proximal to the wrist between tendons of FDS and FCR.
- It then passes deep to fléxor retinaculum into the palm.
- In forearm, it is accompanied by median branch of anterior interrosseous artery.

Branches

Muscular: All superficial flexors except FCU.

Anterior interrosseous nerve - supplies all deep flexors except FDP ulnar half.

Palmar cutaneous branch

- Starts just proximal to flexor retinaculum, pierces it or deep fascia and supplies the skin of the palm.

Median nerve in the hand

- Proximal to flexor retinaculum the nerve is latera to tendons of FDS, but further distally it lies between the retinacula and tendons in carpal tunnel.
- Distal to retinacula, nerve enlarges and flattens.

Branches

Muscular: Just distal to flexor retinaculum-turns round the distal border of the retinaculum to lie just superficial to flexor pollicis brevis.

- Gives branches to thenar muscles and first and second lumbricals.

Sensory

- Divides usually into 4-5 digital branches.
- Passes distally deep to superficial palmar arch and its digital vessels, at first anterior to long flexor tendons
- Supply thumb and two and half digits
- In digits, nerves run distally behind long flexor tendons, out side their fibrous sheath, and anterior to digital arteries.

Diagnosis

1. Loss of flexion of wrist, loss of flexion at PIP and DIP joints.

2. Loss of opponens function
3. Loss of sensations in radial three and half digits.

Management

Initial management is same AS described previously for any other nerve. However author is of opinion that immediate opponensplasty should be done with management of nerve.

Opponensplasty

Muscles used

The muscles usually used are:

- Plamaris longus (Camitz transfer)
- Half palmaris longus (Author's procedure).
- Extensor indicis proprius(Hueber)
- Abductor digiti Minimi(Royle thompson)
- Flexor digitorum superficialis (Bunnel)

Pulley

The pulley is the important structure in opponensplasty AS due to complex movements involved in opponensplasty. Thumb opposition is best restored by transfers that run subcutaneously across the palm, parallel to the abductor pollicis brevis tendon. So all true extrinsic opponensplasties must pass around a stout fixed pulley in the region of the pisiform on the ulnar border of the wrist. This is true for muscles of flexor compartemt.

For muscles from extensor compartment, the passage around ulnar border of the wrist or through interosseous membrane works AS pulley.

Insertion

- Single insertion
- Dual insertion

Dual insertion

It works two functions -Usually active opposition and either passive stabilization of the MP Joint or restriction of inter phalangeal joint flexion, which is beneficial in combined median and ulnar paralysis.

However, tendon transfers are most efficient when they perform only one active function.

Single insertion

Bunnel-drill hole in the dorsoulnar aspect of the base of the thumb in proximal phalanx.

- Tendon of abductor pollicis longus on the radial aspect of the thumb MP Joint.
- Abductor pollicis brevis tendon.
- Dorsal MP Joint capsule or thumb extensor expansion.

General principles of tendon transfer

1. Elective tendon transfer should not be performed in presence of unhealed wound.

2. Full passive joint motion should be restored before tendon transfer.

3. The transfer should not pass through areas of scar tissue or under skin grafts. Further more, surgical incisions should not be placed directly over the transfer.

4. Whenever possible, cutaneous sensibility should be restored before tendon transfer.

5. The transferred muscle should be under voluntary control and must have an independent function.

6. Reinnervated muscle should be used, only if no other muscle is available.

7. Transfer should be straight. If required , no more

than one pulley should be used.

8. Synergism between muscles's original and new action facilitates rehabilitation.

Preoperative treatment of: contractures in relation with opponensplasty

Established soft tissue contractures must be corrected either before or during opponensplasty, because no opponensplasty has sufficient strength to improve the preoperatve passive range of opposition.

First web space contractures are generally due to contractures of the skin and deep fascia on it's extensor surface, contracture of the dorsal capsule of the trapeziometacarpal joint, which restricts opposition but permits abduction, is detected by careful clinical examination.

Method

- Dorsal web space incision.
- Fascia over adductor pollicis and first dorsal interrosseous muscle is released and dorsal web space defect resurfaced with a skin graft or flap.
- Capsular contracture of trapeziometacarpal joint is released through small incision over the base of the joint. However in most of the cases trapeziectomy is needed.

Extensor indicis proprius transfer

Incision

A short incision is made over the index finger MP joint and the EIP tendon is divided immediately proximal to extensor hood

Procedure

After the EIP tendon is harvested, a long incision is made on dorsoulnar aspect of the distal forearm, and the extesnor indicis tendon is delivered into this wound, and it and its muscle are freed of soft tissue attachments on the distal third of the forearm. Next small incision is made in the pisiform area and on the dorsoradial aspect of the MP joint of thumb.

- A wide subcutaneous tunnel is then developed from the extensor surface of the forearm to thumb incision, passing around the ulnar border of the wrist and across the palm.
- The extensor tendon is passed through this tunnel superficial to FCU, otherwise there is risk of ulnar nerve being compressed.

Distal attachment in isolated median palsy, attach to the abductor pollicis brevis tendon with wrist in thirty degrees flexion and thumb in maximum opposition. In combined median and ulnar palsy, transfer is attached in sequence to abductor pollicis brevis tendon, MP joint capsule, and EPL tendon over the proximapl phalanx. This attachment restricts IP joint flexion and thus allows FPL to flex the MP joint more effectively and substitute for paralyzed flexor pollicis brevis.

Postoperatively

The thumb is immobilized with wrist in flexion and thumb in opposition.

Chapter-18
Common Peroneal Nerve

Anatomy

- Arises from sciatic.
- Descends obliquely along the popliteal fossa to the lateral side of the head of fibula, medial to the biceps femoris tendon and lying between its tendon and the lateral head of gastrocnemius.
- Curves lateral to fibular neck, deep to the peroneus longus and divides into superficial and deep peroneal nerves.

Deep peroneal

- Begins at the common peroneal bifurcation.
- Passes obliquely forwards deep to the EDL in front of interosseous membrane, reaching to the anterior tibial artery in proximal third of the leg, descending with it to the ankle.
- Divides into lateral and medial terminal branches.
- Medial terminal branch runs distally on the dorsum of the foot lateral to the dorsalis pedis artery and supplies first web space and adjacent side of the toes.

Superficial peroneal

- Begins at the common peroneal bifurcation.
- At first deep to the peroneus longus, passes antero-

inferiorly between peronei and EDL to pierce the deep fascia in the leg's distal third, where it divides into lateral and medial branches.

- Between muscles it supplies peronei.
- The medial branch passes anterior to the ankle, dividing into two dorsal digital nerves, one supplying the medial side of hallux, and the other the adjacent side of second and the third toes.
- The smaller lateral branch traverses the dorsum of the foot laterally, divides into dorsal digital branches which supply contiguous sides of 3rd to fifth toes, also supplying the skin of the ankle's lateral aspect continuing with sural nerve.

Muscles supplied

- All the extensor muscles.
- Peronei.

Problem

Foot drop

Managment

1. Nerve injuries should be dealt AS other nerves.
2. Muscle paralysis is dealt with TP transfer.

TP transfer

Anatomy

- Lies between Flexor hallucis longus and Flexor digitorum longus.
- Most deeply placed flexor.
- Medial part of the muscle is attacged to interrosseous membrane and shaft of tibia.
- Lateral part is attached to posterior fibular surface.

- Tendon passes deep to that of FDL sharing a groove behind the medial malleolus, but both are enclosed in a separate synovial sheaths.
- Passes deep to flexor retinaculum.
- Enters the foot and divides into superficial and deep division
- Superficial division is attached to the navicular tuberosity, from which fibres continue to the inferior surface of the medial cuneiform.
- Deeper tendon ends on intermdeiate cuneiform and bases of 2nd/4th metatarasals.

Action

Invertor and planter flexor of the foot.

Incisions

- In foot two or three small incisions on the dorsal aspect proximally for retrieving tibialis posterior, extensor hallucis longus, tibialis anterior, and extensor digitorum.
- In lower leg on the medial aspect, a curved incision to pull the muscle in the leg where it is divided in two slips Standard) or three slips Author).
- After division, all the slips are rerouted on the dorsum of the foot and are anastomosed with extensor tendons.
- POP cast is given to foot being kept in dorsiflexion for three weeks

Chapter-19

Volkman's Contracture and Compartment Syndrome

Compartment syndrome is defined AS a condition in which the circulation within a closed compartment is compromised by an increase in pressure within the compartment resulting in tissue death. Pressure interferes with the circulation of the blood to the muscles and nerves in the compartment, and if untreated may result in Volkman's contracture

Causes

- Crush injuries
- Prolonged external compression,
- Internal bleeding
- Excessive exercises
- Burns
- Intraarterial injections.

Diagnosis

- Pain is the most consistent symptom
- Forearn is tense with swelling
- Sensibility of fingertips is diminished
- Passive extension of the fingers increases the pain.
- Radial pulse may or may not be palpable.

Management

Fasciotomy

Established Volkman's contracture

The earliest changes usually involve the flexor digitorum profundus muscles in the middle third of the forearm.

Tsuge has classified the contracture in three types

Mild

In this condition single muscle groups, particularly wrist flexors are involved.

Treatment

Dynamic splinting and physiotherapy .May need muscle tendon lengthening.

Moderate

A moderate contracture usually involves all the flexors of the forearm.

Treatment

- Neurolysis of nerves.
- Excision of any fibrotic muscle mass.
- Muscle slide
- If no useful ampiltude of movements of the fingers has been retained tendon transfers.

Severe

Involves both flexors and extensors.

Treatment

- Excision of all fibrosed mass of muscles.
- Neurolysis of nerves
- Muscle slide
- Tendon transfers
- Free muscle transfer

Muscle sliding operation for flexors for established Volkman's contracture

Incision

It extends along the course of ulnar nerve from a point a hands breadth above the medial epicondyle to the wrist.

Procedure

Ulnar nerve is identified.

It is freed upto the point of entry in forearm between two heads of flexor carpi ulnaris.

Medial intermuscular septum is excised.

Upper margin of flexor muscles is identified at the elbow and the plane between the flexors and brachialis muscle is developed

Then the flexor muscle mass is detached from medial epicondyle, capsule of the elbow joint, and the coronoid process of ulna

- The common aponeurosis between flexor carpi ulnaris and extensor carpi ulnaris is then incised over the subcutaneous border of ulna in its upper third
- The dissection proceeds proximally to detach the ulnar head of flexor carpi ulnaris and so the dissection becomes continuous with the previous one
- This allows the ulnar nerve to be transposed anterior to the medial epicondyle as the flexor mass slides distally.
- The disection is now carried distally along the subcutaneous border of ulna AS for AS the wrist
- The flexor mass is elevated in an extraperitoneal fashion from the ulna and retracted towards the radius

- The interrosseous memebrane is identified and all the muscles attached are separated from the anterior and anterolateral aspect of radius
- At the end radius and ulna are exposed on their anterior aspect, distally AS far AS pronator quadratus and proximally in the radius AS far AS the supinator muscles
- Great care should be taken all the times to avoid the damage to the main vessles and the medial nerve at the elbow.

When the detachment is complete it should be possible to place the wrist in 30 degree of dorsiflexion and extend the fingers and the thumb completely.

Immobilization

The limb is immobilized in a plaster slab maintaining the wrist in dorsiflexion, and the fingers semiflexed at IP Joints but extended at MP Joints.

Functioning muscle transplantation

In many cases the muscles are so much damaged that for proper functioning healthy muscles are needed. In today's era of microsurgery when facilities of microsurgery are much advanced, functioning muscle transfer is the answer in such cases.

The functioning free muscle transplantation involves the transfer of a skeletal muscle from one site to another by microneurovascular techniques. An undamaged motor nerve in the recipient site is sutured to the motor nerve of the transplanted muscle to achieve reinnervation and active muscle contraction. Circulation is maintained by microvascular anastomosis of the artery and vein of the transplanted muscle to suitable vessels in the recipient site.

Before going for operation ascertain:

1. Good range of passive joint motion
2. Proximal joint stability and balance.
3. Good skin cover.
4. Good bed for tendon gliding.

Technique

The description of the operative technique applies to the forearm although the principles are the same for any site of extremity transplantation

Muscles used

The usual muscles used are pectoralis major,latissimus dorsi and gracilis.Gracilis is usually preferred because of its functioning capability for adequately replacing the forearm flexor musculature.

Harvesting of gracilis muscle

Anatomy

Gracilis arises by a thin aponeurosis from the medial margin of the ischiopubic rami and the adjacent body of the pubis. It is widest and thickest superiorly and narrows AS it descends, to end AS a rounded tendon, which crosses the medial side of knee between sartorius and semitendinosus to be inserted into the upper medial tibia.

Arterial supply conforms to the type 2 pattern with a primary dominant pedicle arising from the profunda femoris artery and entering the muscle on its deep surface at the junction of the upper one -third with the lower two thirds. This vessel measures between 1-2 mm in diameter and is accompanied by paired venae comitantes. A secondary pedicle arises from the superficial femoral artery, passes between adductor longus and brevis, gives off a branch to adductor magnus and finally enters gracilis in its lower third. Few minor vessels also supply gracilis at its origin from the medial circumflex femoral artery.

Main vessel of gracilis arises from profunda femoris and passes medially between adductor longus and adductor brevis supplying them and ending in gracilis. The artery enters about 8 cm beneath the pubic crest.

Nerve supply

Nerve supply is from obturator nerve which descends through the obturator foramina superiorly, deep to adductor longus muscle on adductor brevis and enters the gracilis muscle on its deep surface at the same level AS vacular hilum.

A branch to adductor longus muscle should be preserved by intraneural dissection back to obturator foramina where the nerve is the divided.

Elevation of muscle

- Patient lies supine.
- Muscle is marked before hand by asking the patient to adduct.
- Incision is made.
- Once the incision is made, anterior border of gracilis is defined inferior to estimated level of vascular pedicle.
- It is retracted from posterior border of adductor longus.
- Neurovascular pedicle is identified at the junction of the upper quarter and lower three quarteres of gracilis and the vessels are traced laterally deep to adducor longus.
- The vessels are traced upto profunda vessels
- The length of the pedicle is approximately 6 cm and the diameter of the vessels at their origin is

usually 2 mm.

- When the garcilis is transferred for reconstruction, it is desirable to preserve AS much AS epimysial tissue AS possible to allow gliding
- Before detaching muscle put silk sutures at regular intervals. At recipient site this interval is to be maintained. This is for maintaining proper tension, otherwise muscle may not function properly.

Transfer

- Any of the recipient vessel and the nerve are dissected.
- Gracilis is transferred and placed with normal tension.
- Proximally it is attached to medial epicondyle
- Distally it is attached to tendons.
- Donor vessel and the nerve are anastomosed with recipient vessels and the nerve.

Chapter-20

Entrapement Neuropathies in the Upper Limb

Nerves of upper limb are at risk at several well- determined sites where they pass through a tunnel or the muscle, or beneath the fibrous band.

The harm may result from direct pressure or from ischemia. Motor fibres are more susceptible to pressure effects. However in mixed nerve sensory disturbances may bring the patient to the doctor.

Differential diagnosis

Other causes of mixed neuropathies should be excluded like: diabetes, cervical spondylosis, syringomyelia, outlet syndrome, multiple sclerosis etc.

Usual compression sites

Radial nerve

At the site where the posterior interrosseous nerve enters or passes through the supinator muscle.

Ulnar nerve

- In the cubital tunnel
- In the hypothenar region

Median nerve

- While passing through pronator teres muscle, under flexor superficial arch

- In carpal tunnel

Radial entrapement neuropathy

Aetiology

The nerve is compressed as it passes under a tendinous medial margin of extensor carpi radialis brevis, through an arcade of Frohse or AS it traverses the supinator muscle. Numerous aetiological agents have been found in this region.

These are enlarged bursa, ganglion, neoplasm and malunited fractures.

Symptoms

- Pain may be a symptom
- The usual complaint is weakness or complete paralysis of the extensor muscles of the digits and abductor pollicis longus with sparing of extensor carpi radialis longus and usually extensor radialis brevis.

Treatment

- Surgical removal of the cause.
- If the disease is advanced and recovery is not achieved, tendon transfer for paralyzed muscles.

Operation

Incision

The incision extends from the lateral epicondyle to the midforearm and lies between the extensor carpi radialis brevis and extensor digitorum communis muscles.

- After incision two groups of muscles *i.e.* brachioradialis, extensor carpi radialis longus and brevis; are separated upto elbow exposing supinator muscle.
- Posterior interrosseous nerve is observed entering

and leaving supinator and fully exposed by dividing the superficial belly of the muscle.

The lesion is dealt with AS already described.

Ulnar nerve in the cubital tunnel.

Aetiology

- Change in shape of cubital tunnel between extension and flexion.
- Secondary to arthritis of the elbow joint, ganglion, neoplasm.
- Cubitus valgus deformity resulting from malunion or nonunion of the fracture.
- Leprosy.

Symptoms

- paresthesia followed by weakness or wasting of the intrinsic muscles

Treatment

- Exploration.
- Cause should be treated.
- Anterior transposition has been advised by few.

The operation

Incision

- A curved 6 cm incision midway between the medial epicondye and the tip of olecranon.
- The arch and the nerve entering the tunnel are exposed.
- Arch is split with blunt ended scissors throughout its length.
- The same incision is extended proximally and distally to a length of 20 cm.
- The ulnar nerve is isolated preserving the muscu-

lar branches.

- The nerve is lifted and the distal part of intermuscular septum is excised to permit easy displacement of the nerve without kinking.
- The common flexor origin from the medial epicondyle is divided nerve being placed anteriorly.
- The muscles are returned to their normal position and sutured.

Ulnar nerve in the hand

Aetiology

The causes causing the compression of ulnar nerve in the hand are:

- ganglion arising from a carpal joint;
- thrombosis of ulnar artery;
- dislocation of the forth and fifth carpometacarpal joint;.
- ligamentous and muscular anomalies and repeated trauma. This condition has been observed in those patients whose occupation requires them to use the tools, which press continuously upon the ulnar side of the hand.

Symptoms

The symptoms are related to selective pressure upon the motor or the sensory branch of the nerve

- Unilateral weakness of ulnar innervated muscles in the absence of other physical signs should alert one to this diagnosis.

Treatment

Indications of surgery

- When there is palpable swelling.
- When there is muscle wasting.

- When the symptoms don't settle.

Incision

The incision extends from 3 cm above the pisiform bone to the middle palmar crease, curving along the lateral border of hypothenar eminence.

The incision is deepened. The roof of the Guyon's canal in incised to expose the nerve and its bifurcation. If the pathology is not immediately clear, the nerve is followed by separating flexor digiti minimi from its origin and dividing opponens.

The palmar course of the motor branch is traced by lifting the flexor tendons forwards.

Median nerve in the forearm

Aetiology

Anterior interosseous nerve is more susceptible to pressure effects than is the main trunk of the median nerve.

The compression may occur in relation to the pronator teres muscle or to an abnormal band distal to this muscle.

Symptoms

- Usually the symptoms are abrupt.
- There is history of lifting a heavy object, or of a vigorous muscular action immediately preceding the paralysis.
- Pain is commonly felt in the upper arm followed by inability to flex the thumb and weakness of the index finger flexion.

Treatment

- Conservative by rest in a sling or cast.
- If the signs of recovery are not observed within 8 weeks exploration is advisable

The operation

Incision

- Follows the curved course from just distal to elbow crease to just beyond the midpoint of the forearm.
- Deep fascia is divided to expose the median nerve lying on the medial side of the brachial vessels.
- The superficial head of the pronator is divided and the arch joining the to heads of superficialis is also divided.

Median nerve in carpal tunnel

Aetiology

Compression of the median nerve within the carpal tunnel can be caused by any condition which diminishes the capacity of the tunnel Like :

- carpal dislocation;
- fracture or arthritis;
- ganglion or neoplasm;
- muscle anomaly;
- thickening of the retinaculum AS in acromegaly;

However common cause is idiopathic due to increased bulk of synovium

Symptoms

Symptoms of primary carpal tunnel syndrome develop slowly and may be brought for many months before advice is sought.

- There is feeling of discomfort or tingling in digits supplied by the median nerve, notably in middle and ring finger-symptoms are more prominent in the night.

Tanzer test

Ask the patient to flex the fingers strongly while the wrist is held in flexion. The action compresses the median nerve against the retinaculum and increases the paresthesia.

Treatment

Conservative

- Night splint in slight extension
- Injection of the steroid in the tunnel.

Operative treatment consists of division of the retinaculum

The operation

- The incision is 4-5 cm long, commencing in the proximal part of the thenar crease and crosses the wrist making a slight curve to the medial side AS it does so.
- Care is taken to avoid the palmar cutaneous branch of the median nerve, division of which can lead to a sensitive neuroma and may be the cause of distress.
- Incision is deepened through the fat until the retinacula is clearly defined
- The retina cula is incised with a knife and the underlying tendons are seen
- Compression of the nerve is noted and internal neurolysis is done if required.
- The internal neurolysis is required if the nerve is thickened and fibrosed.

